Take Control of Your Heart Health

How to Reverse Heart Disease and Improve Cardiac Health

Susan D. Brier

Table of Contents

Introduction

Heart disease is one of the leading causes of death in the United States, accounting for about 1 in 4 deaths. With the rise in obesity, diabetes and other lifestyle-related diseases, the number of people affected by heart disease is on the rise. While there is no cure for heart disease, there are ways to reduce its progression and even reverse it.

This is done by making lifestyle changes, such as a healthier diet, regular exercise, stress management and quitting smoking. Through a combination of these strategies, it is possible to reverse the damage caused by heart disease and improve heart health.

The first step to reversing heart disease is to adopt a heart-healthy diet. This includes reducing the amount of saturated fat, sodium and cholesterol in your diet, while increasing the amount of fruits, vegetables, whole grains and low-fat dairy products. It is also important to limit the amount of processed foods and fast foods that are high in saturated fat and sodium. Eating a diet rich in fiber, such as beans and legumes, can help reduce cholesterol levels in the blood. It is also important to limit or avoid alcohol, as it can raise blood pressure and contribute to heart disease.

In addition to dietary changes, regular exercise is also essential for reversing heart disease. Attempt to engage in moderate-intensity physical activity most days of the week for at least 30 minutes. This can include walking, jogging, swimming, biking or any other activities that get the heart rate up and make you breathe faster. Exercise not only helps to reduce cholesterol levels, but also helps to reduce stress and improve overall health.

Stress management is another important factor for reversing heart disease. Chronic stress can contribute to high blood pressure and other risk factors for heart disease. Finding ways to reduce and manage stress, such as through meditation, yoga, deep breathing or other relaxation techniques, can help to reduce these risks. It is also important to get plenty of sleep and to find ways to cope with stress in healthy ways.

Finally, it is essential to quit smoking to reverse heart disease. Smoking increases the risk of heart attack, stroke and other cardiovascular diseases. Quitting smoking can help to reduce these risks and improve overall heart health.

By making these lifestyle changes, it is possible to reverse the damage caused by heart disease and improve heart health. It is important to consult with a physician before making any changes to your diet or exercise routine. With the right plan and support, it is possible to reduce the risk of heart disease and enjoy a healthier, longer life.

Chapter 1: Understanding Heart Disease

Heart disease is a general term used to describe a range of conditions that affect the heart. It is a leading cause of death in the United States and affects millions of Americans. The most common type of heart disease is coronary artery disease, which affects the blood vessels that supply the heart muscle with oxygen-rich blood. Other types of heart disease include arrhythmias, heart valve problems, cardiomyopathy, congenital heart defects, and diseases of the blood vessels, such as aneurysms.

Understanding how heart disease develops and progresses is essential for prevention and treatment. It begins with the buildup of plaque in the arteries, which is caused by high cholesterol, high blood pressure, diabetes, smoking, and other risk factors. Plaque is a hard, waxy substance composed of cholesterol, calcium, and other substances. As the plaque accumulates, it narrows the arteries and reduces the flow of oxygen-rich blood to the heart muscle. Angina or chest pain may result from this. Over time, the plaque can rupture or break off, forming a clot that can completely block the artery and cause a heart attack.

It is important to identify risk factors that may contribute to the development of heart disease. These include high cholesterol, high blood pressure, diabetes, smoking, being overweight or obese, physical inactivity, and unhealthy eating habits. Treating and managing these risk factors can help reduce the risk of heart disease.

Lifestyle changes, such as eating a healthy diet and getting regular exercise, can also help reduce the risk of heart disease. Eating a diet that is low in saturated and trans fat, cholesterol, and sodium and high in fiber, fruits, and vegetables is recommended. Regular physical activity can help lower blood pressure and cholesterol levels and improve overall heart health. Quitting smoking is also essential for reducing the risk of heart disease.

In addition to lifestyle modifications, medications may be prescribed to treat heart disease and reduce the risk of heart attack and stroke. These medications may include aspirin, beta-blockers, ACE inhibitors, and statins. These medications can help lower blood pressure, reduce cholesterol, and reduce the risk of blood clots that can lead to heart attack and stroke.

Understanding heart disease is essential for prevention and treatment. Knowing the risk factors and making lifestyle changes, such as eating a healthy diet, getting regular exercise, and quitting smoking, are key for reducing the risk of heart disease. Medications may also be prescribed to help treat and manage the condition. With proper treatment and management, heart disease can be prevented and controlled.

Heart disease is a serious and potentially life-threatening condition, but it can be prevented and managed with the right lifestyle changes, medications, and medical treatment. Understanding the risk factors, making the necessary lifestyle changes, and seeking medical care are important for reducing the risk of heart disease. Making these changes can not only help prevent heart disease, but also improve overall health and quality of life.

Chapter 2: Risk Factors for Heart Disease

Heart disease is a serious health issue, and is the leading cause of death in the United States. Knowing the risk factors associated with heart disease can help you understand your risk and take steps to reduce it.

Some risk factors for heart disease are non-modifiable, meaning they cannot be changed. These include age, sex, and family history. Age is a major risk factor, as the risk of developing heart disease increases with age. Men have a greater risk than women, and those with a parent or sibling with heart disease are also at higher risk.

Other modifiable risk factors include lifestyle, diet, and exercise. Smoking is a major risk factor and is linked to narrowing of the arteries, which can lead to a heart attack. Eating a diet high in saturated fat, trans fat, and cholesterol, can increase your risk of developing heart disease. Not exercising regularly, being overweight or obese, and having a sedentary lifestyle can also increase your risk.

High blood pressure, cholesterol, and diabetes are medical conditions that can increase your risk of heart disease. High blood pressure puts extra strain on your heart and can damage the arteries. High cholesterol can cause fatty deposits to build up in your arteries, narrowing them and blocking blood flow. Diabetes can cause damage to the blood vessels, leading to a higher risk of heart disease.

Heart disease is a major cause of death and disability throughout the world. It is a term used to refer to a wide range of diseases that affect the heart, including coronary artery disease, arrhythmias, heart defects, and heart failure. While some heart conditions are inherited, many are caused by lifestyle factors, such as poor diet, lack of physical activity, smoking, and excessive alcohol consumption.

Understanding the various causes of heart disease can help to identify risk factors, reduce the risk of developing the disease, and improve outcomes for those who do have heart disease.

Diet

A poor diet is one of the primary causes of heart disease. Eating too much saturated fat, trans fat, and cholesterol can increase blood cholesterol levels, leading to an increased risk of coronary artery disease. Eating too much salt can also increase blood pressure, further increasing the risk of coronary artery disease. Eating too much sugar can also lead to weight gain, which can increase the risk of developing heart disease.

Lack of Physical Activity

Regular physical activity can help to reduce the risk of heart disease by strengthening the heart and improving circulation. However, a lack of physical activity can increase the risk of developing heart disease.

Those who are physically inactive are more likely to be overweight, which can increase the risk of developing heart disease. Additionally, those who are not physically active are more likely to have high blood pressure, high cholesterol levels, and diabetes, all of which can increase the risk of heart disease.

Smoking

Smoking is one of the leading causes of heart disease. Smoking increases the risk of developing coronary artery disease, as well as other cardiovascular diseases. Smoking increases the risk of developing atherosclerosis, a condition in which plaque builds up in the arteries, narrowing them and reducing the flow of blood. As a result, a heart attack or stroke may occur.

Additionally, smoking increases the risk of developing arrhythmias, or irregular heartbeats, which can lead to sudden cardiac death.

Excessive Alcohol Consumption

Excessive alcohol consumption can increase the risk of developing heart disease. Alcohol can increase blood pressure and lead to arrhythmias, as well as increase the risk of developing atrial fibrillation, a type of irregular heartbeat.

Additionally, excessive alcohol consumption can increase the risk of developing cardiomyopathy, or damage to the heart muscle, which can lead to heart failure.

Stress

Heart disease risk can rise as a result of stress. Stress can increase blood pressure and heart rate, which can increase the risk of coronary artery disease. Additionally, stress can lead to unhealthy coping mechanisms, such as overeating and smoking, which can further increase the risk of heart disease.

Understanding the various causes of heart disease can help to identify risk factors and reduce the risk of developing the disease. A healthy diet, regular physical activity, and avoiding smoking and excessive alcohol consumption can help to reduce the risk of heart disease. Additionally, reducing stress and learning healthy coping mechanisms can help to reduce the risk of developing heart disease.

It's important to understand your risk factors for heart disease, and take steps to reduce them. Eating a healthy diet, exercising regularly, quitting smoking, and managing stress can all help reduce your risk. If you have any medical conditions, it's important to work with your healthcare provider to manage them. Taking these steps can help you reduce your risk of developing heart disease and improve your overall health.

Chapter 3: Diet and Lifestyle Changes to Reverse Heart Disease

Diet and lifestyle changes are essential for reversing heart disease. A heart-healthy diet consists of eating a variety of vegetables and fruits, whole grains, healthy fats, and lean proteins. Eating foods that are high in fiber and low in saturated fats, trans fats, and sodium can help reduce cholesterol and lower your risk of heart disease. Limiting unhealthy habits like smoking, excessive drinking, and not getting enough physical activity also play a role in reversing heart disease.

It is important to note that diet and lifestyle changes will take time to have an effect on heart disease. It is important to be patient and consistent in making these changes to see the best results. Working with a healthcare professional to create an individualized plan to reverse heart disease can be beneficial.

Heart disease is a serious and common condition that affects millions of people around the world. Fortunately, there are many steps individuals can take to reduce their risk of developing heart disease or to reverse existing heart disease. Making changes to diet and lifestyle are two of the most effective ways to improve heart health.

Diet

Eating a healthy, balanced diet is a key factor in reversing heart disease. Reducing or eliminating foods high in saturated fat, trans fat, and cholesterol, such as red meat, full-fat dairy products, and processed foods, is recommended. Eating a diet high in fruits and vegetables, lean proteins, and whole grains can help reduce cholesterol levels, lower blood pressure, and improve overall heart health.

Lifestyle

In addition to dietary changes, making lifestyle changes can have a positive impact on heart health. Regular physical activity is important, as it helps to maintain a healthy weight and reduce cholesterol levels. Reducing stress and quitting smoking are also recommended, as they can reduce the risk of developing heart disease. Additionally, getting enough sleep and managing alcohol consumption can also help improve heart health.

Making changes to diet and lifestyle are not always easy, but they can have a major impact on heart health. Taking the time to adjust one's diet and lifestyle can help reverse heart disease and reduce the risk of developing heart disease in the future.

In addition to eating a healthy diet and exercising regularly, other lifestyle changes can help reverse heart disease. These include managing stress, quitting smoking, and limiting alcohol consumption. Making these changes can help reduce your risk of developing heart disease and improve your overall cardiovascular health.

Chapter 4: Exercise and Physical Activity for Cardiac Health

Exercise and physical activity are key components of a healthy lifestyle and are essential for maintaining cardiac health. Regular physical activity helps to reduce high blood pressure, improve cholesterol levels, and reduce the risk of cardiovascular disease, stroke, and other chronic diseases. In addition, exercise and physical activity can help to strengthen the heart, improve circulation, and reduce stress.

It is important to check with your doctor before starting any exercise program. Your doctor can provide guidance on the best exercise program for your individual needs. Additionally, it is important to start slowly, gradually increasing the intensity and duration of your activity. It is also important to warm up before exercise and cool down afterwards. Finally, it is important to stay hydrated and to monitor your heart rate during exercise.

Cardio exercise, such as walking, jogging, cycling, swimming, and stair climbing, are all excellent choices for cardiovascular conditioning. Strength training, such as weight lifting and isometric exercises, can help to strengthen the heart muscles, improve balance, and reduce the risk of falls.

In addition to exercise, it is important to make healthy lifestyle choices that promote cardiac health. Eating a balanced diet, maintaining a healthy weight, avoiding smoking, and limiting alcohol consumption can all help to reduce the risk of cardiovascular disease. It is also important to practice stress management techniques, such as yoga and meditation, to help reduce stress and anxiety.

For those with existing heart problems, exercise can help to improve cardiac function and reduce the risk of complications such as heart attack and stroke. Exercise can also help reduce cholesterol levels, which can reduce the risk of coronary artery disease.

In general, adults should aim for at least 150 minutes of moderate-intensity aerobic activity per week, such as walking, swimming, or cycling. A combination of aerobic and strength training exercises, such as weight lifting or yoga, is also recommended.

To maintain optimal cardiac health, it is important to practice good habits such as eating a healthy, balanced diet and avoiding smoking. It is also important to get regular checkups and follow recommended medical advice. Exercise and physical activity can help to enhance overall cardiac health and reduce the risk of serious illnesses.

Chapter 5: Stress Management and Emotional Well-Being

Stress management and emotional well-being are essential aspects of heart health. Stress and emotional distress can increase the risk for heart disease, as well as worsen symptoms for those who already have it. Chronic stress can cause changes in the body that can lead to high blood pressure, chest pain, and an irregular heartbeat.

Therefore, it is important to learn how to manage stress and maintain emotional well-being in order to reduce the risk of heart disease. The ability to manage stress and emotions effectively is linked to better adherence to lifestyle and medication changes, as well as lower levels of inflammation and improved physical health.

Stress is a normal part of life, but when it becomes excessive or unmanaged, it can take a toll on the body and mind. Stress can come from both internal and external sources, and is typically experienced as a feeling of being overwhelmed or out of control. In the long term, chronic stress can lead to physical and emotional health problems, including high blood pressure, heart disease, depression, and anxiety.

When it comes to emotional well-being, it is important to recognize the importance of self-care and the need to take time for yourself. This can include activities such as mindfulness, yoga, and regular physical activity. It is important to make sure you are getting enough restful sleep.

When it comes to managing stress, it is important to recognize your own stress triggers and develop strategies to cope with them. This may include breathing exercises, journaling, or talking to a trusted friend or professional.

Another important way to maintain emotional well-being is to foster strong relationships with family and friends. It is also important to recognize the importance of social support, social support can help reduce stress levels and improve overall mental health. No matter how strong and independent you may be, having a strong support system is essential.

Additionally, engaging in activities that bring pleasure, such as hobbies or spending time outdoors, is important for emotional well-being.If you are struggling with stress or emotional well-being, reach out to those you trust and build a support system.

Also, it is important to be mindful of your diet. Eating a healthy, well-balanced diet can help to reduce stress levels and promote emotional well-being. Eating a diet rich in fruits and vegetables, lean proteins, healthy fats, and whole grains can help to maintain a healthy heart and reduce the risk of heart disease.

Lastly, it is important to seek help if needed. Talking to a mental health professional or talking to a trusted friend can help reduce stress levels and provide emotional support. The goal is to manage stress and maintain emotional well-being in order to reduce the risk of heart disease.

In summary, managing stress and emotional well-being is essential for maintaining a healthy heart. Taking time for yourself, developing stress-coping strategies, creating a support system, and eating a healthy diet can all help to reduce the risk of heart disease.

By implementing these strategies, individuals can reduce their risk of heart disease and improve their overall well-being.

Chapter 6: Medications and Procedures to Treat Heart Disease

Medications

The most common medications used to treat heart disease are those that reduce the risk of developing heart disease, such as statins, ACE inhibitors, beta blockers, and aspirin. Statins help to reduce the amount of cholesterol in the blood, ACE inhibitors help to lower blood pressure, and beta blockers help to reduce the heart rate.

Aspirin helps to prevent blood clots and can reduce the risk of stroke. Other medications such as diuretics and calcium channel blockers may also be prescribed to treat heart disease.

Medications:

1. *ACE inhibitors*: ACE inhibitors (angiotensin-converting enzyme inhibitors) are a type of medication used to treat high blood pressure, heart failure, and other conditions. They work by widening blood vessels and reducing the amount of work the heart has to do to pump blood.

2. *Beta-blockers*: Beta-blockers are a type of medication used to treat high blood pressure, angina, irregular heartbeats, and other conditions. They work by blocking certain hormones that constrict blood vessels, allowing blood to flow more easily.

3. *Calcium channel blockers*: Calcium channel blockers are a type of medication

used to treat high blood pressure, angina, irregular heartbeats, and other conditions. They work by blocking the movement of calcium into cells, which helps relax the muscles of the heart and blood vessels.

4. *Diuretics*: Diuretics are a type of medication used to treat high blood pressure and other conditions. They work by increasing the amount of water and salt that is eliminated through urine, which reduces the amount of fluid in the body and helps reduce blood pressure.

Procedures

Heart procedures can also be used to treat heart disease. Coronary angioplasty and stenting are two common procedures used to treat coronary artery disease. These procedures involve the insertion of a catheter into the blocked artery and the placement of a tiny metal tube (stent) to keep the artery open. Other procedures such as coronary artery bypass grafting, angiography, and pacemaker implantation are also used to treat heart disease.

In addition to medications and procedures, lifestyle modifications can also help to treat heart disease. These modifications include eating a healthy diet, exercising regularly, quitting smoking, and reducing stress. Other treatments, such as cardiac rehabilitation and stress management, can also help to reduce the risk of heart disease.

Procedures:

1. *Coronary artery bypass grafting (CABG):* CABG is a type of surgery used to treat blocked or narrowed coronary arteries. During the procedure, healthy arteries or veins from other areas of the body are grafted onto the blocked coronary artery to improve blood flow to the heart.

2. *Percutaneous coronary intervention (PCI):* PCI is a type of procedure used to treat blocked or narrowed coronary arteries. During the procedure, a catheter is inserted into the blocked artery and a balloon is inflated to widen the artery and improve blood flow to the heart.

3. *Implantable cardiac defibrillator (ICD):* An ICD is a device that is implanted in the

chest to detect and treat dangerous heart rhythms. The device monitors the heart and can deliver an electrical shock to restore a normal heart rhythm if necessary.

4. *Pacemaker*: A pacemaker is a device that is implanted in the chest to help regulate the heart rhythm. The device monitors the heart and can send electrical signals to the heart to help maintain a normal rhythm.

Those are some of the medications and procedures used to treat heart disease. It is important to talk to your doctor to determine which treatment is best for you.

Conclusion

Although the battle against heart disease is far from ending, advancements have been made in our knowledge of and ability to treat this deadly and sneaky condition. We have been able to lower the incidence and mortality of heart disease thanks to a greater understanding of its causes, risk factors, and therapies.

Although there is no one specific treatment for heart disease, there are steps anyone can do to lower their risk and live a healthy life. We must continue to urge people to lead healthy lifestyles while promoting awareness of and education about heart disease. We can only make a difference in the battle against heart disease by banding together.

An overview of heart disease, including its causes and therapies, is given in this book. We've looked at the risk factors and spoken about methods to lower them. We have examined the existing therapies, including prescription drugs and way-of-life adjustments. Finally, we discussed the value of taking care of oneself and how to lead a healthy lifestyle.

Even if there is no single treatment for heart disease, the likelihood of getting the illness and dying from it can still be decreased. We can lower the incidence and mortality of heart disease by being aware of the risk factors, adopting a healthy lifestyle, and utilizing the available therapies.

We must keep advancing heart disease education and awareness while enticing individuals to lead healthy lifestyles. We can only make a difference in the fight against heart disease by banding together.

www.ingramcontent.com/pod-product-compliance
Lightning Source LLC
Chambersburg PA
CBHW051717250726
48653CB00007B/3070